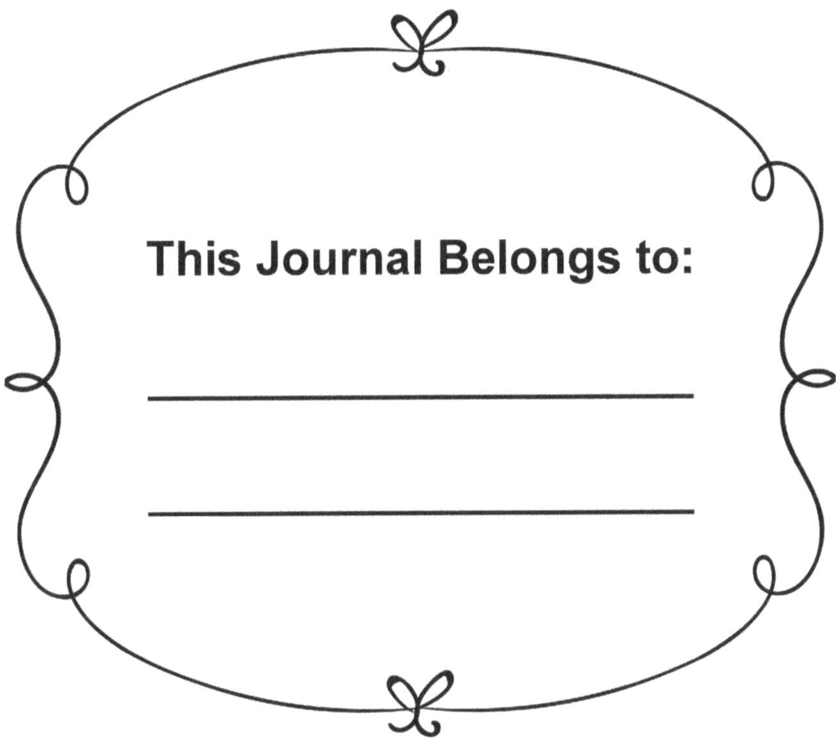
This Journal Belongs to:

How to Use this Bible Verse Journal

Notice this Bible Verse Journal Is for Women to Write In.
Each Blank Page is for you to document God's comfort to you through specific Bible verses found throughout God's Word. The useful free-form format includes lined blank pages to make journaling easy.

- Praise be to the God and Father of our Lord Jesus Christ. He is the Father who is full of mercy, the God of all comfort. (2 Corinthians 1:3 ERV - Easy to Read Version)

Meditate on Quotes from Scripture Promising the Peace of God:
Christian women have been comforted throughout the ages by the promises found in God's Word. While all Bible study is helpful, this journaling experience is upon Bible verses that provide comfort to women experiencing pain and heartache.

Include Praise to God in Your Journaling As God Comforts You:
The Apostle Paul encouraged his readers to focus upon praising God in the midst of pain and heartbreak. As you document how God is comforting you through scripture, you will want to do so in the context of giving praise to God.

As you journal, may these most loved passages of Scripture give you hope, peace, and joy, resulting in "Praise to the God and Father of our Lord Jesus Christ. . .the God of all comfort."

Notice how you are prompted to praise and sing in response to God's comfort.

- "Praise the LORD! He has heard my prayer for mercy. The LORD is my strength and shield. I trusted Him with all my heart. He helped me, so I am happy. I sing songs of praise to Him." (Psalms 28:6-7 ERV)

- "Praise the LORD! Give thanks to the LORD because He is good! His faithful love will last forever! No one can describe how great the LORD really is. No one can praise Him enough." (Psalms 106:1-2 ERV)

Share God's Comfort with Others Who Are Going Through Trials and Difficulties:
- "Praise be to the God and Father of our Lord Jesus Christ. He is the Father who is full of mercy, the God of all comfort. He comforts us every time we have trouble so that when others have trouble, we can comfort them with the same comfort God gives us. (2 Corinthians 1:3-4 ERV);

- "We must hold on to the hope we have, never hesitating to tell people about it. We can trust God to do what He promised."
- (Hebrews 10:23 ERV)

Leave a Legacy of Faith by Journaling God's Comfort to You:
Sharing how God comforted you through scripture is a way for you to impact future generations. They too will experience pain and heartbreak in life. By keeping journals that focus on your spiritual journey, you can help them face their own trials and challenges.

So Tell Your Story of the God of All Comfort by Journaling:
Yes, you could write using apps and programs tied to whatever the latest technology offers. Yet even the most up-to-date tool is soon obsolete! But a written journal can be passed on to future generations.

Journaling is the closest method that we can use to tell the miracles of God, one generation to another.

- We have heard the story, and we know it well. Our fathers told it to us. And we will not forget it. Our people will be telling this story to the last generation. We will all praise the LORD and tell about the amazing things he did. (Psalms 78:3-4 ERV)

"I pray that God will open your minds to see his truth. Then you will know the hope that he has chosen us to have. You will know that the blessings God has promised his holy people are rich and glorious." (Ephesians 1:18 ERV)

"Our descendants will serve him. Those who are not yet born will be told about him. Each generation will tell their children about the good things the Lord has done." (Psalms 22:30-31 ERV)

"He made an agreement with Jacob. He gave the law to Israel. He gave the commands to our ancestors. He told them to teach the law to their children." (Psalms 78:5 ERV)

"Praise be to the God and Father of our Lord Jesus Christ. In Christ, God has given us every spiritual blessing in heaven." (Ephesians 1:3 ERV)

"In Christ, he chose us before the world was made. He chose us in love to be his holy people--people who could stand before him without any fault." (Ephesians 1:4 ERV)

"I will tell you a story. I will tell you about things from the past that are hard to understand. We have heard the story, and we know it well. Our fathers told it to us." (Psalms 78:2-3 ERV)

"And we will not forget it. Our people will be telling this story to
the last generation. We will all praise the LORD and tell about
the amazing things he did." (Psalms 78:4 ERV)

"May those in faraway countries remember the LORD and come back to him. May those in distant lands worship him, because the LORD is the King. He rules all nations." (Psalms 22:27-28 ERV)

"The people have eaten all they wanted and bowed down to worship him. Yes, everyone will bow down to him-- all who are on the way to the grave, unable to hold on to life." (Psalms 22:29 ERV)

"Great blessings belong to those who don't listen to evil advice, who don't live like sinners, and who don't join those who make fun of God. Instead, they love the LORD'S teachings and think about them day and night." (Psalms 1:1-2 ERV)

"So they grow strong, like a tree planted by a stream-- a tree that produces fruit when it should and has leaves that never fall. Everything they do is successful." (Psalms 1:3 ERV)

"But I trust in your unfailing love, my heart rejoices in your salvation. I will sing the LORD's praise, for he has been good to me." (Psalms 13:5-6 NIV)

"My steps have held to your paths, my feet have not stumbled. I call on you, my God, for you will answer me, turn your ear to me and hear my prayer." (Psalms 17:5-6 NIV)

"The LORD is my rock, my fortress and my deliverer, my God is my rock, in whom I take refuge, my shield and the horn of my salvation, my stronghold." (Psalms 18:2 TNIV)

"I called to the LORD, who is worthy of praise, and I have been saved from my enemies." (Psalms 18:3 TNIV)

"God is the one who gives me strength. He clears the path I need to take. He makes my feet as steady as those of a deer. Even on steep mountains he keeps me from falling."
(Psalms 18:32-33 ERV)

"The law of the LORD is perfect, refreshing the soul. The statutes of the LORD are trustworthy, making wise the simple." (Psalms 19:7 TNIV)

"The precepts of the LORD are right, giving joy to the heart. The commands of the LORD are radiant, giving light to the eyes." (Psalms 19:8 TNIV)

"Let the words of my mouth, and the meditation of my heart, be acceptable in thy sight, O LORD, my strength, and my redeemer." (Psalms 19:14 KJV)

"LORD, show me your ways. Teach me how to follow you."
(Psalms 25:4 NIrV)

"Guide me in your truth. Teach me. You are God my Savior. I put my hope in you all day long." (Psalms 25:5 NIrV)

"LORD, remember your great mercy and love. You have shown them to your people for a long time."
(Psalms 25:6 NIrV)

"Don't remember the sins I committed when I was young. Don't remember how often I refused to obey you. Remember me because you love me. LORD, you are good." (Psalms 25:7 NIrV)

"The LORD is honest and good. He teaches sinners to walk in his ways." (Psalms 25:8 NIrV)

"LORD, I have done many wrong things. But I ask you to forgive them all to show your goodness." (Psalms 25:11 ERV)

"When people choose to follow the LORD, he shows them the best way to live." (Psalms 25:12 ERV)

"I always look to the LORD for help. Only he can free me from my troubles." (Psalms 25:15 ERV)

"I am hurt and lonely. Turn to me, and show me mercy. Free me from my troubles. Help me solve my problems. Look at my trials and troubles. Forgive me for all the sins I have done." (Psalms 25:16-18 ERV)

"Every word of God is flawless. He is a shield to those who take refuge in Him." (Proverbs 30:5 WEB)

"So faith comes by hearing, and hearing by the Word of God."
(Romans 10:17 WEB)

"God makes people right through their faith in Jesus Christ. He does this for all who believe in Christ. Everyone is the same." (Romans 3:22 ERV)

"All have sinned and are not good enough to share God's divine greatness." (Romans 3:23 ERV)

"They are made right with God by his grace. This is a free gift. They are made right with God by being made free from sin through Jesus Christ." (Romans 3:24 ERV)

"Being therefore justified by faith, we have peace with God through our Lord Jesus Christ, through whom we also have our access by faith into this grace in which we stand. We rejoice in hope of the glory of God." (Romans 5:1-2 WEB)

"But here is how God has shown his love for us. While we were still sinners, Christ died for us." (Romans 5:8 NIrV)

"If you openly say, 'Jesus is Lord' and believe in your heart that God raised him from death, you will be saved. Yes, we believe in Jesus deep in our hearts, and so we are made right with God. And we openly say that we believe in him, and so we are saved." (Romans 10:9-10 ERV)

"Therefore I urge you, brothers, by the mercies of God, to present your bodies a living sacrifice, holy, acceptable to God, which is your spiritual service." (Romans 12:1 WEB)

"Don't be conformed to this world, but be transformed by the renewing of your mind, so that you may prove what is the good, well-pleasing, and perfect will of God."
(Romans 12:2 WEB)

"Trust the LORD completely, and don't depend on your own knowledge. With every step you take, think about what he wants, and he will help you go the right way."
(Proverbs 3:5-6 ERV)

"Now may the God of hope fill you with all joy and peace in believing, that you may abound in hope, in the power of the Holy Spirit." (Romans 15:13 WEB)

"Come to me, all you who labor and are heavily burdened, and I will give you rest. Take my yoke upon you, and learn from me, for I am gentle and humble in heart, and you will find rest for your souls. For my yoke is easy, and my burden is light." (Matthew 11:28-30 WEB)

"But as many as received him, to them he gave the right to become God's children, to those who believe in his name." (John 1:12 WEB)

"The Word became flesh, and lived among us. We saw his glory, such glory as of the one and only Son of the Father, full of grace and truth." (John 1:14 WEB)

"For God so loved the world, that he gave his one and only Son, that whoever believes in him should not perish, but have eternal life." (John 3:16 WEB)

"Again, therefore, Jesus spoke to them, saying, 'I am the light of the world. He who follows me will not walk in the darkness, but will have the light of life.'" (John 8:12 WEB)

"Don't let your heart be troubled. Believe in God. Believe also in me. In my Father's house are many homes. If it weren't so, I would have told you. I am going to prepare a place for you." (John 14:1-2 WEB)

"If I go and prepare a place for you, I will come again, and will receive you to myself, that where I am, you may be there also." (John 14:3 WEB)

"I am the vine. You are the branches. He who remains in me, and I in him, the same bears much fruit, for apart from me you can do nothing." (John 15:5 WEB)

"If you remain in me, and my words remain in you, you will ask whatever you desire, and it will be done for you." (John 15:7 WEB)

"I have told you these things, that in me you may have peace. In the world you have trouble, but cheer up! I have overcome the world." (John 16:33 WEB)

"If anyone speaks, let it be as it were the very words of God. If anyone serves, let it be as of the strength which God supplies, that in all things God may be glorified through Jesus Christ, to whom belong the glory and the dominion forever and ever. Amen." (1 Peter 4:11 WEB)

"Humble yourselves therefore under the mighty hand of God, that he may exalt you in due time, casting all your worries on him, because he cares for you." (1 Peter 5:6-7 WEB)

"But the fruit of the Spirit is love, joy, peace, patience, kindness, goodness, faith, gentleness, and self-control. Against such things there is no law." (Galatians 5:22-23 WEB)

"For it is by grace you have been saved, through faith--and this is not from yourselves, it is the gift of God-- not by works, so that no one can boast." (Ephesians 2:8-9 NIV)

"Now to him who is able to do exceedingly abundantly above all that we ask or think, according to the power that works in us, to him be the glory in the assembly and in Christ Jesus to all generations forever and ever. Amen." (Ephesians 3:20-21 WEB)

"For you were once darkness, but are now light in the Lord. Walk as children of light, for the fruit of the Spirit is in all goodness and righteousness and truth, proving what is well pleasing to the Lord." (Ephesians 5:8-10 WEB)

"Finally, be strong in the Lord, and in the strength of his might. Put on the whole armor of God, that you may be able to stand against the wiles of the devil." (Ephesians 6:10-11 WEB)

"For to me to live is Christ, and to die is gain."
(Philippians 1:21 WEB)

"Have this in your mind, which was also in Christ Jesus, who, existing in the form of God, didn't consider equality with God a thing to be grasped, but emptied himself, taking the form of a servant, being made in the likeness of men." (Philippians 2:5-7 WEB)

"Therefore God also highly exalted him, and gave to him the name which is above every name, that at the name of Jesus every knee should bow, of those in heaven, those on earth, and those under the earth, and that every tongue should confess that Jesus Christ is Lord, to the glory of God the Father." (Philippians 2:9-11 WEB)

"Brothers and sisters, I know that I still have a long way to go.
But there is one thing I do: I forget what is in the past and try
as hard as I can to reach the goal before me."
(Philippians 3:13 ERV)

"I keep running hard toward the finish line to get the prize that is mine because God has called me through Christ Jesus to life up there in heaven." (Philippians 3:14 ERV)

"'Rejoice in the Lord always!' Again I will say, 'Rejoice!'"
(Philippians 4:4 WEB)

"In nothing be anxious, but in everything, by prayer and petition with thanksgiving, let your requests be made known to God. And the peace of God, which surpasses all understanding, will guard your hearts and your thoughts in Christ Jesus." (Philippians 4:6-7 WEB)

"A whole generation will serve him -- they will tell the next generation about the sovereign Lord. They will come and tell about his saving deeds -- they will tell a future generation what he has accomplished." (Psalms 22:30-31 NET.)

"O God, you have taught me since I was young, and I am still declaring your amazing deeds." (Psalms 71:17 NET.)

"Even when I am old and gray, O God, do not abandon me, until I tell the next generation about your strength, and those coming after me about your power." (Psalms 71:18 NET.)

"Praise the LORD! I thank the LORD with all my heart in the assembly of his good people. The LORD does wonderful things, more than anyone could ask for."
(Psalms 111:1-2 ERV)

"And before the world was made, God decided to make us his own children through Jesus Christ. This was what God wanted, and it pleased him to do it." (Ephesians 1:5 ERV)

"I keep asking that the God of our Lord Jesus Christ, the glorious Father, may give you the Spirit of wisdom and revelation, so that you may know him better." (Ephesians 1:17 NIV)

"And you will know that God's power is very great for us who believe. It is the same as the mighty power he used to raise Christ from death and put him at his right side in the heavenly places." (Ephesians 1:19-20 ERV)

"Remember your promise to me, your servant. It gives me hope. You comfort me in my suffering, because your promise gives me new life." (Psalms 119:49-50 ERV)

"Now our Lord Jesus Christ himself, and God our Father, who loved us and gave us eternal comfort and good hope through grace, comfort your hearts and establish you in every good work and word." (2 Thessalonians 2:16-17 WEB)

"Christ encourages you, and his love comforts you. God's Spirit unites you, and you are concerned for others." (Philippians 2:1 CEV)

"Blessed are those who mourn, for they shall be comforted."
(Matthew 5:4 WEB)

"Praise be to the God and Father of our Lord Jesus Christ. God has great mercy, and because of his mercy he gave us a new life. This new life brings us a living hope through Jesus Christ's resurrection from death." (1 Peter 1:3 ERV)

"Keep yourselves in God's love, looking for the mercy of our Lord Jesus Christ to eternal life." (Jude 1:21 WEB)

"Let's therefore draw near with boldness to the throne of grace, that we may receive mercy, and may find grace for help in time of need." (Hebrews 4:16 WEB)

"But God is rich in mercy, and he loved us very much. We were spiritually dead because of all we had done against him. But he gave us new life together with Christ." (You have been saved by God's grace.)" (Ephesians 2:4-5 ERV)

"Yes, God's riches are very great! His wisdom and knowledge have no end! No one can explain what God decides. No one can understand his ways." (Romans 11:33 ERV)

"The things he does are great and glorious! There is no end to his goodness. He does amazing things so that we will remember that the LORD is kind and merciful."
(Psalms 111:3-4 ERV)

"Wisdom begins with fear and respect for the LORD. Those who obey him are very wise. Praises will be sung to him forever." (Psalms 111:10 ERV)

"LORD, be kind to us. We have waited for your help. Give us strength every morning. Save us when we are in trouble."
(Isaiah 33:2 ERV)

"I don't care about my own life. The most important thing is that I finish my work. I want to finish the work that the Lord Jesus gave me to do -- to tell people the Good News about God's grace." (Acts 20:24 ERV)

"When he came and saw the grace of God, he rejoiced and encouraged them all to remain true to the Lord with devoted hearts." (Acts 11:23 NET.)

"But I do not consider my life worth anything to myself, so that I may finish my task and the ministry that I received from the Lord Jesus, to testify to the good news of God's grace."
(Acts 20:24 NET.)

"For I am not ashamed of the Good News of Christ, because
it is the power of God for salvation for everyone who believes
-- for the Jew first, and also for the Greek."
(Romans 1:16 WEB)

"Only let your way of life be worthy of the Good News of Christ, that, whether I come and see you or am absent, I may hear of your state, that you stand firm in one spirit, with one soul striving for the faith of the Good News." (Philippians 1:27 WEB)

"Give thanks to the LORD and call out to him! Tell the nations what he has done!" (1 Chronicles 16:8 ERV)

"Sing to him -- sing praises to him. Tell about the amazing things he has done. Be proud of his holy name. You followers of the LORD, be happy!" (1 Chronicles 16:9-10 ERV)

"Be proud of his holy name. You followers of the LORD, be happy!" (1 Chronicles 16:10 ERV)

"Depend on the LORD for strength. Always go to him for help. Remember the amazing things he has done. Remember his miracles and his fair decisions." (1 Chronicles 16:11-12 ERV)

"Remember the amazing things he has done. Remember his miracles and his fair decisions." (1 Chronicles 16:12 ERV)

"Give thanks to the LORD, because he is good and because his gracious love is eternal!" (1 Chronicles 16:34 ISV)

"Call out, 'Save us, God, you who delivers us! Gather us and rescue us from the nations! We will thank your holy name and rejoice as we praise you!'" (1 Chronicles 16:35 ISV)

"Praise the LORD God of Israel, who lives from eternity to eternity! Then all of the people shouted 'Amen!' and praised the LORD." (1 Chronicles 16:36 ISV)

"I praise the LORD because he is good. I praise the name of the LORD Most High." (Psalms 7:17 ERV)

"I will make your name to be remembered in all generations. Therefore the peoples shall give you thanks forever and ever." (Psalms 45:17 WEB)

"So we, your people and sheep of your pasture, will give you thanks forever. We will praise you forever, to all generations." (Psalms 79:13 WEB)

"A song of praise for the Sabbath. It is good to praise the LORD. God Most High, it is good to praise your name. It is good to sing about your love in the morning and about your faithfulness at night." (Psalms 92:1-2 ERV)

"A song of thanks. Earth, sing to the LORD! Be happy as you serve the LORD! Come before him with happy songs!"
(Psalms 100:1-2 ERV)

"Know that the LORD is God. He made us, and we belong to him. We are his people, the sheep he takes care of."
(Psalms 100:3 ERV)

"Enter his gates with thanksgiving and his courts with praise, give thanks to him and praise his name. For the LORD is good and his love endures forever -- his faithfulness continues through all generations." (Psalms 100:4-5 NIV)

"Give thanks to the LORD and call out to him! Tell the nations what he has done! Sing to him -- sing praises to him. Tell about the amazing things he has done." (Psalms 105:1-2 ERV)

"Be proud of his holy name. You followers of the LORD, be happy! Depend on the LORD for strength. Always go to him for help. Remember the amazing things he has done. Remember his miracles and his fair decisions." (Psalms 105:3-5 ERV)

"Praise the LORD! Give thanks to the LORD because he is good! His faithful love will last forever! No one can describe how great the LORD really is. No one can praise him enough." (Psalms 106:1-2 ERV)

"Search me, God, and know my heart. Try me, and know my thoughts. See if there is any wicked way in me, and lead me in the everlasting way." (Psalms 139:23-24 WEB)

"Call on me in prayer and I will answer you. I will show you great and mysterious things which you still do not know about." (Jeremiah 33:3 NET.)

"Rejoice always. Pray without ceasing. In everything give thanks, for this is the will of God in Christ Jesus toward you." (1 Thessalonians 5:16-18 WEB)

"God is our protection and source of strength. He is always ready to help us in times of trouble. So we are not afraid when the earth quakes and the mountains fall into the sea." (Psalms 46:1-2 ERV)

"My Lord, you are good and merciful. You love all those who call to you for help. LORD, hear my prayer. Listen to my cry for mercy. I am praying to you in my time of trouble. I know you will answer me." (Psalms 86:5-7 ERV)

"LORD, teach me your ways, and I will live and obey your truths. Help me make worshiping your name the most important thing in my life." (Psalms 86:11 ERV)

"So trust in the LORD and do good. Live on your land and be dependable. Enjoy serving the LORD, and he will give you whatever you ask for. Depend on the LORD. Trust in him, and he will help you." (Psalms 37:3-5 ERV)

"I have been young, and now am old, yet I have not seen the righteous forsaken, nor his children begging for bread." (Psalms 37:25 WEB)

"Indeed, the LORD is the One who will keep on walking in front of you. He'll be with you and won't leave you or abandon you, so never be afraid and never be dismayed." (Deuteronomy 31:8 ISV)

"Remember, I commanded you to be strong and brave. Don't be afraid, because the LORD your God will be with you wherever you go." (Joshua 1:9 ERV)

"May the LORD bless you and keep you." (Numbers 6:24 ERV)

"May the LORD smile down on you and show you his kindness. May the LORD answer your prayers and give you peace." (Numbers 6:25-26 ERV)

"May the Lord direct your hearts into God's love, and into the perseverance of Christ." (2 Thessalonians 3:5 WEB)

"May the Lord who gives peace give you peace at all times and in every way. May the Lord be with all of you."
(2 Thessalonians 3:16 NIrV)

"The LORD is my strength and my reason for singing. He saved me!" (Psalms 118:14 ERV)

"This is the day the LORD has made. Let us rejoice and be happy today! The people say, "Praise the LORD! The LORD saved us!" (Psalms 118:24-25 ERV)

"Lord, you are my God, and I thank you. My God, I praise you! Praise the LORD because he is good. His faithful love will last forever." (Psalms 118:28-29 ERV)